frazely

Paul's Diary

German Easy Reader - Beginner (A1-A2)

written by *Carolin Baller*

By purchasing this book, you support independent publishing.

Thank you.

www.frazely.c....

Meet Paul

Paul leads a normal and happy life, but there are things that stress him out. While on vacation, he learns about minimalism. Could that be something for him…?

Read about this little experiment in his diary full of useful vocabulary and expressions!

Who is this book for?

Designed to be the first book you ever read in German!
It is written with beginner learners of German (A1 - A2 level) in mind, and contains:

- Only basic vocabulary
- Short sentences
- Context to facilitate understanding
- Full translation

What's in this book?

✓ Over 40 chapters

Over 40 short chapters written specifically to enhance your language learning. It will help you understand more from the context and immerse yourself in the world of Paul.

✓ Simple, yet engaging

This book uses simple vocabulary and expressions, and that's exactly what you need when you start learning a language.

✓ Side-by-side translation of the full text

Each chapter includes a complete translation. Sentences are numbered, enabling you to effortlessly locate the corresponding English phrase. Enjoy the pleasure of reading without the need for a dictionary.

Who are the authors?

Hi there, fellow German enthusiast!

We are Frazely - a small start-up comprised of language lovers on a mission to create useful, engaging, high-quality language learning materials.

We firmly believe that language learning can be both **enjoyable and effective**. If you're tired of boring textbooks and complex grammar rules, welcome to the Frazely family!

We sincerely hope you'll enjoy reading this book and wish you every success in your German language journey.

Lots of love,

Frazely Team

PS: We would love to hear from you! Feedback, questions, and even complaints (though we hope there aren't any...) are all welcome at hello@frazely.com.

Contents

1. Packen

1 Samstag, 10. August

2 Hurra, ich fahre morgen in den Urlaub!

3 Ich freue mich schon! 4 Aber halt, ich bin noch nicht so weit. 5 Ich muss noch packen!

6 Mein Koffer ist noch leer. 7 Los geht's!

8 Ich gehe also in mein Schlafzimmer. 9 Ich stehe vor dem Schrank. 10 Was soll ich nur mitnehmen? 11 Was brauche ich? 12 Ich sehe meine T-Shirts, meine Hosen, meine Socken... 13 Ich habe so viel Kleidung!

14 Was soll ich nur mitnehmen?! 15 Ich kann mich nicht entscheiden! 16 Oh, das macht keinen Spaß...

1. Packing

1 Saturday, August 10th

2 Hooray, I'm going on vacation tomorrow!

3 I'm really looking forward to it!

4 But wait, I'm not ready yet.

5 I still have to pack!

6 My suitcase is still empty.

7 Let's go!

8 I go into my bedroom.

9 I stand in front of the wardrobe.

10 What should I take with me?

11 What do I need?

12 I see my t-shirts, my pants, my socks....

13 I have so many clothes!

14 What should I take with me?!

15 I can't decide!

16 Ugh, this is no fun...

2. Ich bin Paul

1 Oh, ich habe mich nicht vorgestellt! 2 Ich bin Paul. 3 Ich bin 26 Jahre alt. 4 Ich wohne in Deutschland. 5 Das hier ist mein Tagebuch. 6 Also, morgen geht es in den Urlaub! 7

Aber ich muss noch packen. 8 Was brauche ich? 9 Ich brauche Kleidung! 10 Welche Kleidung brauche ich? 11 Und welchen Koffer soll ich nehmen? 12 Groß oder klein?

13 Und ich brauche meinen Ausweis.

14 Aber, oje, wo ist er nur? 15 Der ist wichtig!

16 Oje, ich bin genervt. 17 So viel Stress!

frazely

2. I'm Paul

1 Oh, I didn't introduce myself!

2 I'm Paul.

3 I'm 26 years old.

4 I live in Germany.

5 This is my diary.

6 So, tomorrow I'm going on vacation!

7 But I still have to pack.

8 What do I need?

9 I need clothes!

10 What clothes do I need?

11 And which suitcase should I take?

12 Big or small?

13 I also need my ID.

14 But, oh dear, where is it?

15 It's important!

16 Oh my, I'm annoyed.

17 So much stress!

3. Urlaub

1 Montag, 12. August

2 Juhu, ich bin jetzt im Urlaub! 3 WIR sind im Urlaub! 4 Ich bin hier mit meinem Freund. 5 Mein Freund heißt Tim. 6 Wir haben viel Spaß. 7 Spanien ist sehr schön. 8 Wir gehen hier gerne essen. 9 Und wir gehen im Meer schwimmen. 10 Ich lese auch gern am Strand. 11 Lesen ist mein Hobby. 12 Welches Buch, fragst du? 13 Ich habe ein neues Buch gekauft. 14 Ich habe es hier in Spanien gekauft. 15 Es gab nicht viel Auswahl auf Deutsch. 16 Wir sind ja hier in Spanien. 17 Aber ich habe dieses Buch

gefunden: 18 **Es geht um Minimalismus.**

3. Vacation

1 Monday, August 12th

2 Yay, I'm on vacation now!

3 WE are on vacation!

4 I'm here with my friend.

5 My friend's name is Tim.

6 We are having lots of fun.

7 Spain is very nice.

8 We eat out here a lot.

9 And we swim in the sea.

10 I also like to read on the beach.

11 Reading is my hobby.

12 What book, you may ask?

13 I bought a new book.

14 I bought it here in Spain.

15 There wasn't much choice in German.

16 We are in Spain after all.

17 But I found this book:

18 It's about minimalism.

4. Spanien ist toll!

1 Warum ich hier ein Buch gekauft habe, fragst du? 2 Ich habe viele Bücher zu Hause in Deutschland. 3 Aber ich konnte kein Buch mitnehmen. 4 Ich hatte keinen Platz mehr im Koffer. 5 Ich habe sogar einen großen Koffer genommen. 6 Aber ich hatte trotzdem keinen Platz! 7 Ich habe zu viel Kleidung mitgenommen. 8 Das brauche ich hier alles gar nicht. 9 Warum ich so viel mitgenommen habe? 10 Weil ich mich nicht entscheiden konnte. 11 Ich habe viel zu viele Dinge...

12 Naja, egal, Spanien ist toll! 13 Wir haben eine gute Zeit hier. 14 Das Wetter ist toll...

15 Ich muss aufhören mit Schreiben. 16 Wir wollen essen gehen!

4. Spain is great!

1 Why did I buy a book here, you may ask?

2 I have lots of books at home in Germany.

3 But I couldn't take a book with me.

4 I had no space left in my suitcase.

5 Even though I took a big suitcase.

6 But I still had no space!

7 I brought too many clothes.

8 I don't need all that here.

9 Why did I take so much with me?

10 Because I couldn't make up my mind.

11 I have way too many things...

12 Anyway, Spain is great!

13 We're having a good time here.

14 The weather is great...

15 I have to stop writing.

16 We are going out to eat!

5. Minimalismus

1 Ich schlafe gleich. 2 Aber ich will noch kurz etwas schreiben. 3 Es geht um das Buch, das ich gerade lese. 4 Das Buch über Minimalismus. 5 Was ist eigentlich Minimalismus? 6 Ich weiß es noch nicht genau. 7 Ich habe erst ein bisschen gelesen. 8 Es ist interessant. 9 Es geht um Geld sparen. 10 Und Dinge wegschmeißen. 11 Es soll gut gegen Stress sein. 12 Und es soll glücklich machen. 13 Kann das wahr sein?! 14 Ich kann das nicht glauben. 15 Naja, ich werde es lesen, dann weiß ich mehr. 16 Gute Nacht, ich schlafe jetzt!

5. Minimalism

1 I'm about to go to sleep.

2 But I want to write something quickly.

3 It's about the book I'm reading.

4 The book about minimalism.

5 What exactly is minimalism?

6 I don't really know yet.

7 I've only read a little bit.

8 It's quite interesting.

9 It's about saving money.

10 And throwing things away.

11 It's supposed to be good for stress.

12 And it's supposed to make you happy.

13 Could that be true?!

14 I find it hard to believe.

15 Well, I'll read it, then I'll know more.

16 Good night, I'm going to sleep now!

6. Zurück in Deutschland

1 Samstag, 24. August

2 Wir sind zurück. 3 Der Urlaub ist vorbei.

4 Ich bin wieder zu Hause. 5 Wie war es in Spanien? 6 Spanien war toll! 7 Es war heiß.

8 Das war schön. 9 Der Strand war auch toll!

10 Ich war im Meer schwimmen. 11 Und ich habe viel gelesen. 12 Ich habe das Buch über Minimalismus gelesen. 13 Ich denke, ich will es versuchen. 14 Ich will minimalistisch leben!

6. Back in Germany

1 Saturday, August 24th

2 We are back.

3 The vacation is over.

4 I'm back home again.

5 How was Spain?

6 Spain was great!

7 It was hot.

8 That was nice.

9 The beach was great too!

10 I swam in the sea.

11 And I read a lot.

12 I read the book about minimalism.

13 I think I want to try it.

14 I want to live a minimalist life!

7. Das Experiment

1 Warum ich das will? 2 Im Buch steht, dass Minimalismus glücklich macht. 3 Ich bin nicht unglücklich! 4 Aber ich will mein Leben verbessern. 5 Ich will mein Leben aufräumen. 6 Ich habe zu viele Dinge! 7 Und wie geht das? 8 Ich weiß nicht genau. 9 Aber ich will es versuchen. 10 Es ist ein Experiment.

11 Soll ich jetzt starten? 12 Nein, heute nicht mehr. 13 Ich bin müde. 14 Und ich mache mir gerade eine Pizza! 15 Die will ich gleich essen! 16 Ich werde morgen starten...

7. The experiment

1 Why do I want to do this?

2 The book says that minimalism makes you happy.

3 I am not unhappy!

4 But I want to improve my life.

5 I want to clean up my life.

6 I have too many things!

7 And how does that work?

8 I don't know exactly yet.

9 But I want to try it.

10 It will be an experiment.

11 Should I start now?

12 No, not today.

13 I'm tired.

14 And I was just making a pizza!

15 I want to eat it right away!

16 I'll start tomorrow...

8. Es geht los!

1 Sonntag, 25. August, am Morgen

2 Heute ist es so weit. 3 Ich werde minimalistisch! 4 Ich mache es! 5 Aber wie beginne ich?

6 Ich hole den Mülleimer. 7 Ich stelle ihn in den Flur. 8 Da kommt rein, was ich wegschmeißen will! 9 Das ist der Plan.

10 Jetzt kann es losgehen! 11 Ich gehe ins Schlafzimmer. 12 Es ist ein kleines Zimmer.

13 Wo soll ich beginnen? 14 Mit dem Schrank? 15 Mit dem Schreibtisch? 16 Mit den Boxen? 17 So viele Dinge sind hier!

18 Mh... erstmal ein Kaffee.

8. Off we go!

1 Sunday, August 25th, in the morning

2 Today is the day.

3 I'm going minimalist!

4 I'm going to do it!

5 But how do I start?

6 I get the bin.

7 I put it in the hallway.

8 Everything I want to throw away goes in there!

9 That's the plan.

10 Now I can get started!

11 I go into the bedroom.

12 It's a small room.

13 Where should I start?

14 With the wardrobe?

15 With the desk?

16 With the boxes?

17 There are so many things here!

18 Hmm... first, a coffee.

9. Oh nein...

1 Sonntag, 25. August, später am Tag

2 Oje, was habe ich getan? 3 Meine Wohnung ist so chaotisch! 4 Alle Schränke sind offen. 5 Der Boden ist voller Sachen. 6 Der Mülleimer ist fast leer. 7 Nur drei alte Stifte sind darin! 8 Und mein Basketball und meine Regenjacke. 9 Ich habe meinen Basketball weggeschmissen. 10 Aber den brauche ich doch! 11 Ich habe morgen Training! 12 Und ich habe meine Regenjacke weggeschmissen. 13 Aber die brauche ich auch noch!

14 Ich bin gestresst. 15 So geht das nicht...

16 Ich muss es anders machen.

9. Oh no...

1 Sunday, August 25th, later in the day

2 Oh dear, what have I done?

3 My apartment is so messy!

4 All the cabinets are open.

5 The floor is full of stuff.

6 The bin is almost empty.

7 There are only three old pens in there!

8 And my basketball and my rain jacket.

9 I've thrown away my basketball.

10 But I need it!

11 I have training tomorrow!

12 And I've thrown away my rain jacket.

13 But I still need that too!

14 I'm stressed.

15 It can't go on like this...

16 I have to do it differently.

10. Der Plan

1 Aber wie? 2 Ich habe eine Idee! 3 Vielleicht kann mir das Buch helfen. 4 Ich suche das Buch. 5 Ich lese. 6 Im Buch steht: 7 <Mache dir einen Plan!> 8 Das ist eine gute Idee! 9 Ich mache mir einen Plan. 10 Ich habe noch eine Woche Urlaub. 11 Jeden Tag will ich ein Zimmer machen. 12 Montag mache ich das Badezimmer. 13 Dienstag mache ich das Schlafzimmer. 14 Mittwoch mache ich das Wohnzimmer. 15 Donnerstag mache ich die Küche. 16 Freitag mache ich den Flur. 17 Dann bin ich fertig. 18 Das ist mein Plan. 19 Das wird einfach, oder nicht?

10. The plan

1 But how?

2 I have an idea!

3 Maybe the book can help me.

4 I'm looking for the book.

5 I read.

6 The book says:

7 <Make a plan!>

8 That's a good idea!

9 I come up with a plan.

10 I still have a week of vacation.

11 I want to do one room a day.

12 Monday I'll do the bathroom.

13 Tuesday I'll do the bedroom.

14 Wednesday I'll do the living room.

15 Thursday I'll do the kitchen.

16 Friday I'll do the hallway.

17 Then I'm done.

18 That's my plan.

19 It'll be easy, won't it?

11. Das Badezimmer

1 Montag, 26. August

2 Ich beginne heute mit dem Badezimmer.

3 Schritt für Schritt! 4 Ich denke, das Badezimmer ist nicht so schwer. 5 Ich habe dort nicht so viele Dinge.

6 Ich gehe ins Badezimmer. 7 Ich habe hier Handtücher und ein paar Boxen mit Dingen.

8 Was will ich behalten? 9 Was kann ich wegschmeißen? 10 Ich beginne mit den Handtüchern. 11 Ich habe jetzt sechzehn Stück. 12 Große und kleine. 13 Das ist zu viel! 14 Wie viele brauche ich? 15 Ich will fünf behalten. 16 Das reicht. 17 Aber welche?

11. Bathroom

1 Monday, August 26th

2 I'm starting with the bathroom today.

3 Step by step!

4 I don't think the bathroom will be hard.

5 I don't have too many things in there.

6 I go into the bathroom.

7 I have towels and a few boxes here.

8 What do I want to keep?

9 What can I throw away?

10 I start with the towels.

11 I now have sixteen of them.

12 Big ones and small ones.

13 That's too many!

14 How many do I need?

15 I want to keep five.

16 That's enough.

17 But which ones?

12. Medikamente

1 Ich suche die schönsten Farben aus.

2 Blau und Grün, zwei kleine, drei große.

3 Ich mache weiter mit den Boxen. 4 Ich finde fünf Nagelscheren, zwei Rasierer und Toilettenpapier. 5 Ich brauche nicht so viele Nagelscheren! 6 Ich schmeiße vier weg.

7 Ich finde einen Lippenstift. 8 Die gehört meiner Ex-Freundin. 9 Wir sind schon seit zwei Jahren nicht mehr zusammen! 10 Die Schminke kommt in den Müll. 11 In einer Box sind Medikamente.

12 Ich schmeiße die alten Medikamente weg.

13 Super, das ist ja richtig einfach heute! 14 Jetzt das Schampoo! 15 Ich habe sechs Flaschen.

16 Ich brauche doch nicht so viele Flaschen!

17 Die meisten sind fast leer. 18 Ich schmeiße

sie weg.

12. Medication

1 I choose the most beautiful colors.

2 Blue and green, two small ones, three large ones.

3 I continue with the boxes.

4 I find five nail scissors, two razors and toilet paper.

5 I don't need so many nail scissors!

6 I throw away four.

7 I find a lipstick.

8 It belongs to my ex-girlfriend.

9 We haven't been together for two years!

10 The lipstick goes in the bin.

11 There's some medication in a box.

12 I throw away the old medication.

13 Great, today it's really easy!

14 Now the shampoo!

15 I have six bottles.

16 I don't need that many bottles!

17 Most of them are almost empty.

18 I throw them away.

13. Das nächste Mal

1 Heute lief es gut. 2 Ich habe das Badezimmer gemacht. 3 Ich habe jetzt viel weniger im Bad. 4 Es ist leerer. 5 Es sieht besser aus. 6 Ich fühle mich gut. 7 Das Badezimmer war einfach.

8 Aber war es richtig, die Shampoos wegzuschmeißen? 9 Da war ja noch Shampoo drin... 10 Ich bin mir nicht sicher.

11 Ich hätte sie leer machen sollen. 12 Ja, ich denke, das wäre besser gewesen. 13 Das ärgert mich ein bisschen. 14 Egal, jetzt ist es zu spät. 15 Beim nächsten Mal mache ich es anders.

frazely

13. Next time

1 Today went well.

2 I did the bathroom.

3 I have a lot less in the bathroom now.

4 It's emptier.

5 It looks better.

6 I feel good.

7 The bathroom was easy.

8 But was it right to throw away the shampoos?

9 There was still shampoo in there...

10 I'm not sure.

11 I should have emptied them.

12 Yes, I think that would have been better.

13 That annoys me a bit.

14 Anyway, it's too late now.

15 I'll do it differently next time.

14. Das Schlafzimmer

1 **Dienstag, 27. August**

2 **Heute geht es weiter.** 3 **Auf dem Plan für heute steht das Schlafzimmer.** 4 **Da ist mein Kleiderschrank.** 5 **Dort habe ich viel Kleidung drin.** 6 **Und da ist mein Schreibtisch.** 7 **Ich habe viele Unterlagen und Papiere dort.** 8 **Es ist viel zu tun.** 9 **Ob das gut geht...?**

10 **Erstmal alles raus!** 11 **Ich nehme alle Kleidungsstücke heraus.** 12 **Sie liegen nun auf dem Boden.** 13 **Es ist sehr viel...** 14 **Mh, vielleicht fange ich doch mit dem Schreibtisch an...**

14. Bedroom

1 Tuesday, August 27th

2 Today we continue.

3 On the plan for today is the bedroom.

4 That's where my closet is.

5 I have a lot of clothes in there.

6 And there's my desk.

7 There are a lot of documents and papers.

8 There's a lot to do.

9 Will that go well...?

10 Let's get everything out first!

11 I take out all the clothes.

12 They are now lying on the floor.

13 It's a lot...

14 Hmm, maybe I'll start with the desk after all...

15. Der Schreibtisch

1 Ich gehe zum Schreibtisch. 2 Auf dem Tisch steht eine Box. 3 In der Box sind Stifte, Radiergummi und Kugelschreiber. 4 Ich leere die Box auf dem Boden aus. 5 Oh, und da ist ja eine Gabel! 6 Hä, was macht eine Gabel hier? 7 Ich bringe sie in die Küche.

8 Ich gehe zurück ins Schlafzimmer. 9 Der Schreibtisch hat eine Schublade. 10 Ich öffne sie. 11 Da ist ganz viel Papier drin.

12 Es sind Rechnungen, Verträge, Briefe...

13 Ich lege alles auf den Boden. 14 Ich beginne das Papier zu sortieren. 15 Oh, ich finde eine Postkarte von Jenny! 16 Die soll an

den Kühlschrank! 17 **Ich schaue weiter durch die Papiere.** 18 **Es sind so viele Zettel...**

15. Desk

1 I head to the desk.
2 On the desk there's a box.
3 In the box are pencils, erasers and pens.
4 I empty the box on the floor.
5 Oh, and there's a fork!
6 Huh, what's a fork doing here?
7 I take it to the kitchen.
8 I go back into the bedroom.
9 The desk has a drawer.
10 I open it.
11 There's a lot of papers in there.
12 There are bills, contracts, letters...
13 I put everything on the floor.
14 I start sorting through the papers.
15 Oh, I find a postcard from Jenny!
16 It should go on the fridge!
17 I keep looking through the documents.
18 There are so many papers...

16. Chaos

1 Ich schaue mich in meinem Schlafzimmer um. 2 Der ganze Boden ist voll mit Dingen. 3 Pullover, Socken, Hosen, Papier, Ordner, Stifte... 4 Oje, was für ein Chaos! 5 Mir wird heiß. 6 Ich muss hier raus! 7 Ich gehe aus dem Schlafzimmer.

8 Ich gehe in die Küche. 9 Ich mache mir einen Kaffee. 10 Oje, das ist viel zu viel! 11 Ich bin total gestresst. 12 Ich will das nicht mehr machen. 13 Aufräumen ist stressig. 14 Minimalismus macht keinen Spaß! 15 Ich glaube, ich gebe auf... 16 Das Experiment ist vorbei!

16. Chaos

1 I look around my bedroom.

2 The whole floor is full of things.

3 Sweaters, socks, pants, papers, folders, pens...

4 Oh dear, what a mess!

5 I'm feeling hot.

6 I have to get out of here!

7 I leave the bedroom.

8 I go into the kitchen.

9 I make myself a coffee.

10 Oh dear, that's just too much!

11 I'm totally stressed.

12 I don't want to do this anymore.

13 Cleaning up is stressful.

14 Minimalism is no fun!

15 I think I'll give up...

16 The experiment is over!

17. Moment mal...

1 Nein, was rede ich da... 2 Ich will aufgeben? 3 Weil ich zu viel habe? 4 Weil es mich stresst? 5 Weil es mir zu viel ist? 6 Das ergibt doch keinen Sinn! 7 Das ist doch unlogisch! 8 Ja, es sind zu viele Sachen. 9 Deswegen MUSS ich es tun! 10 Nur dann kann es besser werden! 11 Morgen ist ein neuer Tag. 12 Morgen will ich weitermachen! 13 Es ist schwer, aber ich kann es schaffen! 14 Schritt für Schritt!

17. Wait a minute...

1 No, what am I talking about...

2 I want to give up?

3 Because I have too many things?

4 Because it's stressing me out?

5 Because it's too much for me?

6 That doesn't make any sense!

7 That's illogical!

8 Yes, there are too many things.

9 That's why I HAVE to do it!

10 Only then can it get better!

11 Tomorrow is a new day.

12 Tomorrow I want to keep going!

13 It's hard, but I can do it!

14 Step by step!

18. Ein neuer Versuch

1 Mittwoch, 28. August, am Morgen

2 Es ist ein neuer Tag. 3 Ich will es weiter versuchen. 4 Ich sehe es ja. 5 Meine Dinge stressen mich. 6 Sogar aufräumen stresst mich. 7 Ich habe zu viele Dinge! 8 Das ist doch nicht gut! 9 So will ich das nicht. 10 So will ich nicht leben. 11 Es soll sich etwas ändern. 12 Ich will mich ändern. 13 Ich will Dinge anders machen. 14 Ich will nicht aufgeben. 15 Ich will es versuchen. 16 Heute werde ich weitermachen. 17 Aber wo mache ich weiter?

18. A new attempt

1 Wednesday, August 28th, in the morning

2 It's a new day.

3 I want to keep trying.

4 It's obvious.

5 My things stress me out.

6 Even cleaning up stresses me out.

7 I have too many things!

8 That's not good!

9 That's not how I want it.

10 I don't want to live like this.

11 I want something to change.

12 I want to change.

13 I want to do things differently.

14 I don't want to give up.

15 I want to try.

16 I will carry on today.

17 But where do I continue?

19. Ein neuer Plan

1 Wo mache ich heute weiter? 2 Eigentlich war für heute das Wohnzimmer geplant.

3 Aber mein Schlafzimmer ist ja noch nicht fertig! 4 Das muss ich erst fertig machen.

5 Das werde ich heute tun. 6 Ich werde meinen Schreibtisch aufräumen. 7 Und ich werde meinen Schrank aufräumen.

8 Aber erst einmal Kaffee! 9 Ich mache mir einen Kaffee. 10 Mit dem Kaffee gehe ich in das Schlafzimmer. 11 Ich sehe das Chaos.

12 Oje, wo fange ich nur an... 13 Mir wird es wieder heiß. 14 Aber stopp, keine Panik!

15 Ich denke daran, was im Buch steht:

16 Schritt für Schritt!

19. A new plan

1 What am I going to do today?

2 Today's plan was actually the living room.

3 But my bedroom isn't finished yet!

4 I have to finish that first.

5 I'll do that today.

6 I'm going to clean up my desk.

7 And I'm going to clean out my wardrobe.

8 But first coffee!

9 I make myself a coffee.

10 I take the coffee into the bedroom.

11 I see the mess.

12 Oh dear, where do I start...

13 I'm getting hot again.

14 But stop, don't panic!

15 I think about what the book said:

16 Step by step!

20. Pullover

1 Ich fange mit den Pullovern an. 2 Ich habe zwanzig Pullover. 3 So viele brauche ich doch nicht. 4 Es sind viel zu viele! 5 Aber welche soll ich behalten? 6 Wie soll ich mich entscheiden? 7 Ich schaue mir die Pullover an.

8 Welchen Pullover trage ich oft? 9 Welchen Pullover trage ich gern? 10 Welcher Pullover ist zu klein? 11 Welcher Pullover ist zu groß?

12 Welcher Pullover ist kaputt? 13 Welche Farbe will ich? 14 Diese Fragen helfen mir.

20. Sweaters

1 I'll start with the sweaters.

2 I have twenty sweaters.

3 I don't need that many.

4 There are way too many!

5 But which ones should I keep?

6 How should I decide?

7 I look at the sweaters.

8 Which sweater do I wear often?

9 Which sweater do I like to wear?

10 Which sweater is too small?

11 Which sweater is too big?

12 Which sweater is damaged?

13 Which color do I want?

14 These questions help me.

21. Das ist zu viel!

1 Auf jeden Fall den schwarzen Pullover.

2 Den trage ich oft. 3 Auf jeden Fall den grauen Pullover. 4 Der ist so weich! 5 Dann noch blau und grün. 6 Das sind schöne Farben! 7 Also behalte ich vier Pullover!

8 Die anderen Pullover lege ich in einen Sack.

9 Jetzt die Hosen. 10 Ich habe fünfzehn Hosen. 11 Das ist zu viel!

12 Welche soll ich behalten?

13 Welche Hose trage ich oft?

14 Welche Hose trage ich gern?

15 Welche Hose ist zu klein?

16 Welche Hose ist zu groß?

17 Welche Hose ist kaputt?

21. That's too many!

1 Definitely the black sweater.

2 I wear it a lot.

3 Definitely the gray sweater.

4 It's so soft!

5 Then there's blue and green.

6 Those are beautiful colors!

7 So I'm keeping four sweaters!

8 I'll put the other sweaters in a bag.

9 Now the pants.

10 I have fifteen pairs of pants.

11 That's too many!

12 Which ones should I keep?

13 Which pants do I wear often?

14 Which pants do I like to wear?

15 Which pants are too small?

16 Which pants are too big?

17 Which pants are damaged?

22. Hosen

1 Es gibt Hosen, die ich noch nie getragen habe. 2 Werde ich sie tragen? 3 Ich denke nach. 4 Ich bin mir nicht sicher. 5 Ach, sie sollen weg! 6 Ich lege sie zu den Pullovern in den Sack. 7 Ich fühle mich gut.

8 Jetzt habe ich noch fünf Hosen. 9 Das ist eine gute Anzahl. 10 Zwei Hosen sind für den Sport. 11 Die brauche ich auch. 12 Ich lege die sieben Hosen in den Schrank. 13 Der Rest der Hosen kommt auch in den Sack.

14 Das lief doch ganz gut! 15 Aber puh, jetzt bin ich müde. 16 Es war anstrengend, so viel nachzudenken! 17 Ich mache eine kleine

Pause.

22. Pants

1 There are pants that I have never worn.

2 Will I ever wear them?

3 I wonder.

4 I'm not sure.

5 Well, they should go!

6 I put them in the bag with the sweaters.

7 I feel good.

8 Now I have five pairs of pants left.

9 That's a good number.

10 Two pairs are for sports.

11 I need those too.

12 I put the seven pants in the closet.

13 The rest of the pants go in the bag too.

14 That went quite well!

15 But phew, now I'm tired.

16 All this thinking was exhausting!

17 I'll take a little break.

23. Socken

1 Es geht weiter. 2 Hosen und Pullover sind fertig. 3 Jetzt mache ich die Socken.

4 Ich sammle alle Socken zusammen.

5 Dann schaue ich mir jede Socke an.

6 Kaputte Socken kommen natürlich weg.

7 Ein paar sehen alt aus. 8 Die kommen auch weg. 9 Ok, das war einfach! 10 Jetzt habe ich noch zwölf Paar Socken. 11 Das ist gut!

12 Ich bin zufrieden.

13 Nun die Unterhosen. 14 Ich schaue mir alle Unterhosen an. 15 Ich habe zehn Unterhosen. 16 Sie sind alle noch gut. 17 Ich will alle behalten.

23. Socks

1 On we go.

2 Pants and sweaters are done.

3 Now I do the socks.

4 I collect all the socks together.

5 Then I look at each sock.

6 Damaged socks are thrown away, of course.

7 A few look old.

8 They must go too.

9 Okay, that was easy!

10 Now I have twelve pairs of socks left.

11 That's good!

12 I'm satisfied.

13 Now the underwear.

14 I look at all the underwear.

15 I have ten pairs of underwear.

16 They are all still good.

17 I want to keep them all.

24. T-shirts

1 Heute will ich die Kleidung fertig machen!

2 Es fehlen noch die T-Shirts. 3 Ich suche alle T-Shirts zusammen. 4 Ich habe zwanzig T-Shirts. 5 Das ist zu viel! 6 Ich schaue mir alle an. 7 Welche will ich behalten? 8 Zwei sind sehr alt. 9 Will ich sie noch tragen? 10 Nein, ich habe sie schon lang genug getragen.

11 Sie kommen in den Müll. 12 Vier T-Shirts trage ich nie. 13 Ich lege sie in einen Sack.

14 Jetzt habe ich noch vierzehn T-Shirts.

15 Zwei rote, vier schwarze, drei graue, ein blaues. 16 Die anderen vier T-Shirts sind für den Sport.

24. T-shirts

1 Today I want to finish the clothes!

2 The T-shirts are still missing.

3 I gather all the T-shirts together.

4 I have twenty T-shirts.

5 That's too many!

6 I look at them all.

7 Which ones do I want to keep?

8 Two are very old.

9 Do I still want to wear them?

10 No, I've already worn them long enough.

11 They go in the bin.

12 I never wear four of the T-shirts.

13 I put them in a bag.

14 I still have fourteen T-shirts.

15 Two red, four black, three gray and one blue.

16 The other four T-shirts are for sports.

25. Geschafft!

1 Mittwoch, 28. August, am Abend

2 Heute war ein guter Tag. 3 Ich habe viel geschafft. 4 Ich habe nicht aufgegeben!

5 Mein Schrank ist jetzt leerer. 6 Und mein Schreibtisch ist aufgeräumt. 7 Es war nicht einfach. 8 Aber ich habe es geschafft! 9 Ich habe nun weniger. 10 Es fühlt sich gut an!

11 Ich bin ein bisschen stolz.

12 Aber was mache ich mit den Sachen in dem Sack? 13 Die, die ich nicht mehr möchte? 14 Soll ich sie wegschmeißen?

15 Mh, das fühlt sich nicht gut an... 16 Ich stelle sie in den Flur. 17 Ich werde mir etwas

überlegen.

25. I did it!

1 Wednesday, August 28th, in the evening

2 Today was a good day.

3 I got a lot done.

4 I didn't give up!

5 My wardrobe is emptier now.

6 And my desk is clean.

7 It wasn't easy.

8 But I did it!

9 I have less now.

10 It feels good!

11 I'm a bit proud.

12 But what do I do with the things in the bag?

13 The ones I no longer want?

14 Should I throw them away?

15 Hmm, that doesn't feel good...

16 I'll put them in the hallway.

17 I'll think about something.

26. Schneller und einfacher

1 Donnerstag, 29. August

2 Ich muss etwas erzählen. 3 Heute Morgen hatte ich einen guten Moment. 4 Ich habe Kleidung für den Tag ausgesucht. 5 Und da habe ich gemerkt: 6 Es ist jetzt einfacher und schneller, Kleidung auszusuchen. 7 Es gab ja nicht viel Auswahl. 8 Ich habe ja jetzt weniger Kleidung im Schrank. 9 Ich habe jetzt noch vier Pullover. 10 In den Farben schwarz, grau, blau und grün. 11 Ich habe mich schnell für meinen schwarzen Pullover entschieden. 12 Für meinen einzigen schwarzen Pullover! 13 Es war eine einfache

Entscheidung. 14 **Das hat mir gefallen.**

15 **Minimalismus ist gar nicht so schlecht!**

16 **Es klappt!**

26. Faster and easier

1 Thursday, August 29th

2 I need to tell you something.

3 Something nice happened this morning.

4 I was picking out clothes for the day.

5 And that's when I realized:

6 It's easier and quicker to choose clothes now.

7 There wasn't much choice.

8 I have fewer clothes in my wardrobe now.

9 I have four sweaters now.

10 In black, gray, blue and green.

11 I quickly decided on my black sweater.

12 My only black sweater!

13 It was an easy decision.

14 I liked that.

15 Minimalism isn't so bad!

16 It works!

27. Das Wohnzimmer

1 Heute mache ich das Wohnzimmer. 2 Es ist ein kleines Wohnzimmer. 3 Wie sieht mein Wohnzimmer aus? 4 Ich habe ein Sofa und ein großes Regal. 5 In dem Regal sind viele Bücher. 6 Und da sind zwei große Boxen mit Dingen.

7 Wo fange ich an? 8 Meine Bücher! 9 Ich schaue mir alle Bücher an. 10 Es sind viele.

11 Es sieht gar nicht minimalistisch aus!

12 Mh, wie viele Bücher muss ich weggeben?

13 Ich mag meine Bücher. 14 Es ist meine Sammlung. 15 Lesen ist mein Hobby. 16 Wie soll ich mich da entscheiden? 17 Mh, ich bin

ein bisschen traurig.

27. Living room

1 Today I'm doing the living room.

2 It's a small living room.

3 What does my living room look like?

4 I have a sofa and a large shelf.

5 There are lots of books on the shelf.

6 And there are two big boxes.

7 Where do I start?

8 My books!

9 I look at all the books.

10 There's a lot of them.

11 It doesn't look minimalistic at all!

12 Hmm, how many books do I need to give away?

13 I like my books.

14 It's my collection.

15 Reading is my hobby.

16 How am I supposed to decide?

17 Uh, I'm a bit sad.

28. CDs

1 Ich ignoriere die Bücher erst einmal. 2 Ich mache jetzt etwas anderes. 3 Ich nehme eine Box aus dem Regal. 4 Da sind meine CDs! 5 Oh, die habe ich so lange nicht gehört! 6 Ich will sie hören! 7 Wo ist mein CD-Player? 8 Ich finde ihn in der Ecke hinter dem Sofa. 9 Da ist ganz viel Staub auf ihm. 10 Ich mache ihn sauber. 11 Ich lege eine CD von the Beatles ein. 12 Ich höre mir die Musik an.

13 Oh, das ist toll! 14 Ich höre mir alle CDs an.

15 Oje, es ist jetzt schon Abend. 16 Ich habe den ganzen Tag Musik gehört!

17 Es gibt noch so viel zu tun!

28. CDs

1 I ignore the books for now.

2 I'll do something else instead.

3 I take a box from the shelf.

4 There are my CDs!

5 Oh, I haven't listened to them for so long!

6 I want to listen to them!

7 Where's my CD player?

8 I find it in the corner behind the sofa.

9 There's a lot of dust on it.

10 I clean it.

11 I put in a CD by the Beatles.

12 I listen to the music.

13 Oh, that's great!

14 I listen to all the CDs.

15 Oh dear, it's already evening.

16 I've been listening to music all day!

17 There's still so much to do!

29. Jenny

1 Am Abend telefoniere ich mit Jenny. 2 Sie ist eine Freundin von mir. 3 Ich kenne sie schon lange. 4 Jenny ist immer lustig, das mag ich.

5 Wir haben über Neuigkeiten aus unserem Leben gesprochen. 6 Ich habe ihr von meinem Urlaub erzählt. 7 Und auch, dass ich Minimalismus ausprobiere. 8 Sie findet das interessant. 9 Aber sie will es selbst nicht machen. 10 Sie denkt, sie kann nicht minimalistisch leben. 11 Und sie will es auch nicht. 12 Sie hat viele Sachen. 13 Und sie mag ihre Sachen. 14 Dinge machen sie glücklich, sagt sie. 15 Ich habe gesagt, dass mich viele Gegenstände manchmal nerven. 16 Das findet

Jenny auch. 17 Für den Urlaub zu packen ist anstrengend! 18 Oder wenn sie aufräumen muss! 19 Dann nervt es...

29. Jenny

1 I talk to Jenny on the phone in the evening.

2 She's a friend of mine.

3 I've known her for a long time.

4 Jenny is always funny, I like that.

5 We talked about what's new in our lives.

6 I told her about my vacation.

7 And that I'm trying out minimalism.

8 She thinks it's interesting.

9 But she doesn't want to try it herself.

10 She doesn't think she can live a minimalist life.

11 And she doesn't want to either.

12 She has lots of things.

13 And she likes her things.

14 Things make her happy, she says.

15 I said that lots of things sometimes annoy me.

16 Jenny thinks that too.

17 Packing for vacation is exhausting!

18 Or when she has to clean up!

19 Then it can get annoying...

30. Schöne Dinge

1 Aber Jenny will trotzdem nichts ändern.

2 Sie mag ihre volle Wohnung mit den ganzen Dingen. 3 Sie sagt, sie findet leere Wohnungen langweilig. 4 Solche Wohnungen sind kalt und ungemütlich, sagt sie. 5 Man braucht doch schöne Dinge im Leben, sagt sie. 6 Schöne Dinge machen glücklich!

7 Darüber muss ich einmal nachdenken...

8 Hat sie recht? 9 Braucht man schöne Dinge? 10 Brauche ICH schöne Dinge?

11 Machen sie glücklich? 12 Welche Dinge finde ich eigentlich schön? 13 Mir fällt da gar

nichts ein... 14 Ich finde Deko nicht wichtig.

15 Und mir ist auch nicht wichtig, wie meine

Möbel aussehen.

30. Beautiful things

1 But Jenny still doesn't want to change anything.

2 She likes her full apartment with all the things.

3 She says she finds empty apartments boring.

4 Such apartments are cold and uncomfortable, she says.

5 You need nice things in life, she says.

6 Beautiful things make you happy!

7 I need to think about that...

8 Is she right?

9 Do you need beautiful things?

10 Do I need beautiful things?

11 Do they make you happy?

12 What things do I actually find beautiful?

13 I can't think of anything...

14 I don't find decoration important.

15 And I don't care what my furniture looks like either.

31. Wichtige Dinge

1 Mh.... aber einen Moment mal! 2 Es gibt Dinge, die mir wichtig sind. 3 Die mir Freude machen. 4 Zum Beispiel meine Bücher. 5 Es ist eine Sammlung. 6 Sie bedeutet mir viel. 7 Ich freue mich, wenn ich die Bücher im Regal sehe. 8 Gibt es noch andere Dinge, die mir wichtig sind? 9 Meine Sportsachen. 10 Diese Dinge will ich behalten. 11 Sie machen mich glücklich, weil ich sie benutzen kann. 12 Aber andere Dinge können weg. 13 Ich will nicht, dass die Dinge mich stressen. 14 Und ich will auch mehr Platz haben! 15 Und viele Dinge sind auch

gar nicht schön... 16 Ich will es also weiter versuchen. 17 Ich will weiter minimalistisch werden!

31. Important things

1 Hmm.... but wait a minute!

2 There are things that are important to me.

3 Things that bring me joy.

4 My books, for example.

5 It's a collection.

6 It means a lot to me.

7 I'm happy when I see the books on the shelf.

8 Are there any other things that are important to me?

9 My sports gear.

10 I want to keep these things.

11 They make me happy because I can use them.

12 But other things can go.

13 I don't want things to stress me out.

14 And I also want to have more space!

15 And many things aren't even that pretty...

16 So I want to keep trying.

17 I want to keep going minimalist!

32. Meine Bücher

1 Freitag, 30. August

2 Ich mache das Wohnzimmer weiter. 3 Das Gespräch mit Jenny hat mir geholfen. 4 Jetzt weiß ich, dass ich die Bücher behalten will! 5 Das freut mich. 6 Aber ich nehme die Bücher trotzdem alle aus dem Regal. 7 Ich mache das Regal und die Bücher sauber. 8 Dann sortiere ich sie nach Themen. 9 Thriller, Biografien, Sachbücher. 10 Toll, jetzt kann ich alles besser finden! 11 Ich öffne die letzte Box. 12 Ich finde noch mehr CDs. 13 Ich lege sie in die andere Box. 14 Da sind nun alle CDs drin. 15 Und oh, was ist das? 16 Ich finde eine große Kerze. 17 Es war ein Geschenk von meiner Mutter. 18 Ich

stelle sie auf den kleinen Wohnzimmertisch.

19 Super, das Wohnzimmer ist fertig!

32. My books

1 Friday, August 30th

2 I continue with the living room.

3 The conversation with Jenny helped me.

4 Now I know that I want to keep the books!

5 That makes me happy.

6 But I take all the books off the shelf anyway.

7 I clean the shelf and the books.

8 Then I sort them by subject

9 Thrillers, biographies, non-fiction.

10 Great, now everything is easier to find!

11 I open the last box.

12 I find even more CDs.

13 I put them in the other box.

14 All the CDs are in there now.

15 And oh, what's that?

16 I find a big candle.

17 It was a gift from my mother.

18 I put it on the small living room table.

19 Great, the living room is finished!

33. Rabatt

1 Ich habe heute eine E-Mail bekommen.

2 Da steht, dass ich Rabatt auf T-Shirts bekomme. 3 Es ist ein großer Rabatt, dreißig Prozent! 4 Das ist viel! 5 Ich war ganz aufgeregt. 6 Ich wollte den Rabatt nutzen.

7 Dann spare ich Geld, richtig? 8 Ich wollte schon zum Laden fahren. 9 Aber dann habe ich mich gestoppt. 10 Erst einmal nachdenken... 11 Brauche ich eigentlich neue T-Shirts? 12 Nein, eigentlich nicht.

13 Ich habe doch genug T-Shirts! 14 Nur weil etwas günstig ist, muss man es ja nicht kaufen. 15 Ich fahre also nicht zum Laden.

16 Man spart am meisten, wenn man gar nichts kauft!

33. Discount

1 I got an e-mail today.

2 It said I got a discount on T-shirts.

3 It's a big discount, thirty percent!

4 That's a lot!

5 I was really excited.

6 I wanted to use the discount.

7 It would save me money, right?

8 I was about to drive to the store.

9 But then I stopped myself.

10 Think first...

11 Do I actually need new T-shirts?

12 No, not really.

13 I have enough T-shirts!

14 Just because something is cheap doesn't mean you have to buy it.

15 So I'm not going to the store.

16 You save the most money if you don't buy anything at all!

34. Die Küche

1 Samstag, 31. August

2 Heute mache ich die Küche. 3 Ich gehe in die Küche. 4 Es ist eine kleine Küche. 5 Ich koche nicht oft. 6 Ich habe nicht so viele Dinge hier, denke ich. 7 Die Küche wird einfach!

8 Ich öffne die Schränke und Schubladen.

9 Oh, ich habe doch einige Dinge hier...

10 Das habe ich gar nicht gedacht! 11 Ich habe nur ein paar kleine Schränke. 12 Aber alle Schränke sind voll! 13 Wo fange ich nur an?! 14 Erst einmal nehme ich alles heraus.

15 Ich lege es auf den Küchentisch. 16 Dann

mache ich alles sauber. 17 Das ist ein erster guter Schritt!

34. Kitchen

1 Saturday, August 31st

2 Today I'm doing the kitchen.

3 I go into the kitchen.

4 It's a small kitchen.

5 I don't cook often.

6 I don't have that many things here, I think.

7 The kitchen will be easy!

8 I open the cupboards and drawers.

9 Oh, I do have a few things here...

10 I didn't think so!

11 I only have a few small cupboards.

12 But all the cupboards are full!

13 Where do I start?

14 First of all, I take everything out.

15 I put it on the kitchen table.

16 Then I clean everything.

17 That's a good first step!

35. Tassen und Teller

1 Nun kommen die Dinge wieder zurück in die Schränke und Schubladen. 2 Wo fange ich an? 3 Ich mache die Tassen. 4 Oh, ich habe fünfzehn Tassen! 5 Das wusste ich gar nicht! 6 Welche mag ich? 7 Welche benutze ich nie? 8 Wie viele brauche ich überhaupt?

9 Ich suche mir fünf Tassen aus. 10 Das reicht. 11 Ich stelle sie in den Schrank.

12 Der Rest kommt weg.

13 Dann geht es weiter. 14 Ich habe drei Teller. 15 Die brauche ich alle. 16 Ich habe eine Pfanne und einen Topf. 17 Diese Dinge kommen in den Schrank.

35. Cups and plates

1 I put things back in the cupboards and drawers.

2 Where do I start?

3 I do the cups.

4 Oh, I have fifteen cups!

5 I didn't even know that!

6 Which ones do I like?

7 Which ones do I never use?

8 How many do I even need?

9 I choose five cups.

10 That's enough.

11 I put them in the cupboard.

12 I put the rest away.

13 Then I move on.

14 I have three plates.

15 I need them all.

16 I have a pan and a pot.

17 These things go in the cupboard.

36. Oma

1 Jetzt das Besteck. 2 Ich habe zehn Löffel, zehn Gabeln und zwei Messer. 3 Nur zwei Messer? 4 Wo sind die anderen Messer hin?

5 Ich sollte mir ein paar neue Messer kaufen...

6 Ich schaue weiter. 7 Ich finde einen kaputten Toaster. 8 Der kann weg! 9 Da sind noch alte Zeitschriften. 10 Die brauche ich auch nicht mehr!

11 Dann finde ich etwas Besonderes: 12 Es ist ein bunter Teller. 13 Den benutze ich nie.

14 Aber Moment, der ist von meiner Oma...

15 Den will ich behalten! 16 Es ist eine

schöne Erinnerung an sie.

36. Grandma

1 Now the cutlery.

2 I have ten spoons, ten forks and two knives.

3 Only two knives?

4 Where did the other knives go?

5 I should buy some new knives...

6 I keep looking.

7 I find a broken toaster.

8 It can go!

9 There are also some old magazines.

10 I also don't need them anymore!

11 Then I find something special:

12 It's a colorful plate.

13 I never use it.

14 But wait, it's from my grandma...

15 I want to keep it!

16 It's a nice memory of her.

37. Jenny denkt an mich

1 Es ist Abend. 2 Jetzt treffe ich mich mit Jenny. 3 Ich freue mich. 4 Wir gehen in ein Restaurant. 5 Wir bestellen unser Essen. 6 Wir reden.

7 Sie erzählt mir: 8 Sie war einkaufen, und da musste sie an mich denken. 9 Ich bin überrascht. 10 Was meint sie? 11 Warum musste sie an mich denken? 12 Sie hat überlegt, ob sie etwas kaufen soll, einen Spiegel. 13 Und da hat sie an mich und den Minimalismus gedacht. 14 Sie hat es dann doch gekauft. 15 Weil sie es schön fand.

16 Ich lache. 17 Ich sage ihr, dass ich das gut

verstehen kann.

37. Jenny thinks of me

1 It's evening.

2 I'm meeting with Jenny.

3 I'm looking forward to it.

4 We go to a restaurant.

5 We order our food.

6 We talk.

7 She tells me:

8 She was out shopping and she had to think of me.

9 I'm surprised.

10 What does she mean?

11 Why did she have to think about me?

12 She was thinking about buying something, a mirror.

13 And then she thought of me and minimalism.

14 And then she still bought it.

15 Because she thought it was beautiful.

16 I laugh.

17 I tell her I totally understand.

38. Die Säcke

1 Sonntag, 1. September

2 Heute mache ich den Flur. 3 Dann ist meine ganze Wohnung fertig! 4 Also ist heute der letzte Tag des Experiments!

5 Ich gehe in den Flur. 6 Da stehen die Säcke mit der Kleidung. 7 Die Kleidung, die ich nicht mehr will. 8 Was soll ich damit machen? 9 Mein Freund Tim hatte eine Idee!

10 Es gibt Läden, da kann man alte Kleidung abgeben. 11 Diese Läden verkaufen gebrauchte Kleidung! 12 Ich finde Tims Idee gut. 13 Da kann ich meine Kleidung abgeben.

14 Dann muss ich die Kleidung nicht

wegwerfen. 15 **Ich bekomme kein Geld dafür, aber das ist ok.** 16 **Der Laden hat heute auf.** 17 **Ich fahre gleich hin.**

38. The bags

1 Sunday, September 1st

2 Today I'm doing the hallway.

3 After that, my whole apartment is done!

4 So today is the last day of the experiment!

5 I go into the hallway.

6 There are the bags of clothes there.

7 The clothes I no longer want.

8 What should I do with them?

9 My friend Tim had an idea!

10 There are stores where you can hand in old clothes.

11 These stores sell second-hand clothes!

12 I think Tim's idea is good.

13 I can hand in my clothes there.

14 Then I don't have to throw the clothes away.

15 I don't get any money for it, but that's okay.

16 The store is open today.

17 I'll go there straight away.

39. Der Flur

1 Die Säcke sind weg. 2 Jetzt habe ich wieder mehr Platz im Flur! 3 Ich freue mich darüber.

4 Nun geht es weiter. 5 Ich schaue mir den Flur an. 6 Hier steht ein kleiner Schrank. 7 In dem Schrank sind meine Schuhe und Jacken. 8 Auf dem Schrank sind meine Koffer. 9 Ich beginne mit den Jacken. 10 Ich schaue mir alle Jacken an. 11 Ich habe drei Jacken. 12 Die erste ist für Regen. 13 Die zweite ist für den Winter, sie ist ganz warm.

14 Die dritte ist für den Herbst und den Frühling. 15 Ich brauche alle drei! 16 Ich behalte also alle. 17 Das war einfach.

39. Hallway

1 The bags are gone.

2 I now have more space in the hallway again!

3 I'm happy about that.

4 Now I move on.

5 I take a look at the hallway.

6 There's a small closet here.

7 My shoes and jackets are in the closet.

8 My suitcases are on top of the closet.

9 I start with the jackets.

10 I look at all the jackets.

11 I have three jackets.

12 The first one is for the rain.

13 The second is for winter, it's really warm.

14 The third is for fall and spring.

15 I need all three!

16 So I'm keeping them all.

17 That was easy.

40. Die Schuhe

1 Es geht mit den Schuhen weiter. 2 Ich nehme alle Schuhe aus dem Schrank heraus. 3 Ich mache sauber. 4 Dann schaue ich mir alle Schuhe an. 5 Ich habe acht Paar Schuhe. 6 Ich habe zwei Paar kaputte, alte Schuhe. 7 Die schmeiße ich weg. 8 Dann bleiben noch übrig: 9 Zwei Sportschuhe und zwei normale Schuhe für den Alltag. 10 Und dann sind da noch ein Paar schicke Schuhe. 11 Und ein paar Stiefel für den Winter.

12 Benutze ich alle? 13 Ja, eigentlich schon.

14 Die schicken Schuhe trage ich selten.

15 Aber ich möchte sie für die nächste Feier behalten. 16 Ich behalte also sechs Paar

Schuhe. 17 Ich stelle sie wieder zurück in den Schrank. 18 Ich bin mit dem Flur fast fertig!

40. Shoes

1 I continue with the shoes.

2 I take all the shoes out of the closet.

3 I clean it.

4 Then I look at all the shoes.

5 I have eight pairs of shoes.

6 I have two pairs of broken, old shoes.

7 I throw them away.

8 Then there are still some left:

9 Two sports shoes and two normal shoes for everyday.

10 And then there's one pair of elegant shoes.

11 And a pair of boots for the winter.

12 Do I use them all?

13 Yes, I actually do.

14 I rarely wear the elegant shoes.

15 But I want to keep them for the next party.

16 So I keep six pairs of shoes.

17 I put them back in the closet.

18 I'm almost done with the hallway!

41. Die Koffer

1 Jetzt noch die Koffer. 2 Ich hole sie vom Schrank runter. 3 Ich habe drei Koffer! 4 Das sind zu viele Koffer. 5 Ich brauche sie nicht alle. 6 Sie haben verschiedene Größen: 7 Klein, mittel und groß. 8 Ich möchte den kleinsten und größten behalten. 9 Was mache ich mit dem dritten Koffer? 10 Ich will ihn nicht wegschmeißen... 11 Es ist ein guter Koffer! 12 Was kann ich tun?

13 Mein Vater! 14 Dem kann ich den Koffer geben! 15 Denn er fährt bald in den Urlaub. 16 Und er braucht noch einen Koffer! 17 Das ist eine gute Lösung.

41. Suitcases

1 Now the suitcases.

2 I get them down from the closet.

3 I have three suitcases!

4 That's too many suitcases.

5 I don't need them all.

6 They're different sizes:

7 Small, medium and large.

8 I want to keep the smallest and largest one.

9 What do I do with the third suitcase?

10 I don't want to throw it away...

11 It's a good suitcase!

12 What can I do?

13 My father!

14 I can give him the suitcase!

15 Because he's going on vacation soon.

16 And he still needs a suitcase!

17 That's a good solution.

42. Ein paar Tipps

1 Sonntag, 1. September, am Abend

2 Tim war da. 3 Wir haben einen Film geschaut und geredet. 4 Es gab auch Pizza.

5 Ich habe sie selbst gemacht!

6 Tim sagte, dass meine Wohnung jetzt anders aussieht. 7 Es gibt mehr Platz. 8 Er findet es besser so. 9 Das hat mich gefreut.

10 Es stimmt, es ist nicht mehr so voll! 11 Mir gefällt es jetzt auch besser. 12 Tim sagte, er will seine Wohnung auch aufräumen.

13 Aber er findet es schwer. 14 Es ist nicht einfach anzufangen. 15 Das kann ich gut verstehen! 16 Ich habe ihm ein paar Tipps

gegeben. 17 **Er sagte, er will es versuchen!**

42. A few tips

1 Sunday, September 1st, in the evening

2 Tim was there.

3 We watched a movie and talked.

4 We also had pizza.

5 I made it myself!

6 Tim said that my apartment looks different now.

7 There's more space.

8 He thinks it's better this way.

9 That made me happy.

10 It's true, it's not so full anymore!

11 I like it better now too.

12 Tim said he wants to clean up his apartment too.

13 But he finds it hard.

14 It's not easy to get started.

15 I totally understand that!

16 I gave him a few tips.

17 He said he wanted to try!

43. Das Ende

1 Es ist Sonntagabend.

2 Ich sitze in meinem Wohnzimmer. 3 Ich trinke einen Tee. 4 Und ich denke nach und schreibe in dieses Tagebuch.

5 Das war mein Experiment mit dem Minimalismus. 6 Ich habe alle Zimmer aufgeräumt. 7 Sind wir am Ende angekommen? 8 Ich schaue mich um. 9 Ich habe jetzt Ordnung. 10 Ich weiß, was ich habe. 11 Ich weiß, wo die Dinge sind. 12 Ich habe nur Dinge, die ich mag oder brauche.

13 Aufräumen ist nun einfacher. 14 Mein Leben ist einfacher geworden. 15 Das gefällt

mir. 16 Ich bin jetzt entspannter.

17 Vielleicht macht Minimalismus wirklich

glücklich.

43. The end

1 It's Sunday evening.

2 I'm sitting in my living room.

3 I'm drinking a cup of tea.

4 And I'm thinking and writing this diary.

5 That was my experiment with minimalism.

6 I cleaned all the rooms.

7 Are we at the end?

8 I take a look around.

9 I have order now.

10 I know what I have.

11 I know where things are.

12 I only have things that I like or need.

13 Cleaning is easier now.

14 My life has become simpler.

15 I like that.

16 I'm more relaxed now.

17 Maybe minimalism really does make you happy.

44. Der nächste Urlaub

1 Ok, noch eine Sache. 2 Ich muss etwas erzählen:

3 Jenny hat mich angerufen. 4 Sie fragt, ob ich Lust auf Urlaub habe. 5 Ja, natürlich habe ich Lust! 6 Sie will im Winter nach Portugal.

7 Das ist eine gute Idee! 8 Ich will mitkommen. 9 Das wird ein Spaß! 10 Ich freue mich schon. 11 Und ich freue mich sogar aufs Packen! 12 Dieses Mal wird es einfacher. 13 Ich habe ja jetzt weniger Dinge.

14 Und dieses Mal habe ich bestimmt noch Platz für ein Buch. 15 Oder auch zwei!

44. The next vacation

1 Well, one more thing.

2 I have to tell you something:

3 Jenny called me.

4 She asked if I would like to go on vacation.

5 Yes, of course I would!

6 She wants to go to Portugal in the winter.

7 That's a good idea!

8 I want to come with her.

9 It's going to be fun!

10 I'm already looking forward to it.

11 And I'm even looking forward to packing!

12 It'll be easier this time.

13 I have fewer things now.

14 And this time I'll definitely have space for a book.

15 Or even two!

How did we do?

Dearest Reader,

Congratulations on making it to the end! We truly hope you've enjoyed this book and found it helpful.

How did we do? Would you like more content like this? What was your favorite part? We'd love to hear your thoughts and hope you'll take a moment to review our book. We read every review with great joy! You can also reach us via email at hello@frazely.com.

PS. **We have some good news!** We are always busy creating more cool content for you! You'll find your next engaging book on our author's page.

frazely

We hope you've enjoyed this book.
Thank you for trusting our publication.

www.frazely.com

www.ingramcontent.com/pod-product-compliance
Lightning Source LLC
Chambersburg PA
CBHW050815250726

48653CB00006B/2236